Acne Cure
The Clear Skin Dietary Treatment - Proven Effective way to Prevent Acne

by Barbara Williams

Introduction

This is probably the most effective acne treatment plan you will ever encounter in your life! We are going to break down top foods, top all natural supplements, and also foods you must not eat diet if you want to get rid of your acne.

One of the main causes of acne is a bad build-up of bacteria in your digestive tract. This book contains proven steps and strategies on how to effectively treat acne by making some dietary changes and following a simple anti-acne diet menu plan.

There book is a comprehensive information on acne, its symptoms, causes and risk factors. Also featured in this book are some minerals, vitamins, herbal and other natural supplements that will further boost the wonderful effects of your anti-acne diet.

1: General Overview of Acne

Acne is a skin disease which develops when the hair follicles become clogged up with dead skin cells and oil. Acne is medically known as acne vulgaris and most commonly develops on the upper body.

Acne can be annoyingly persistent and distressing. Acne lesions heal gradually and when one seems to start healing, others seem to develop. Depending on its severity, this skin condition may lead to scarring of the skin and emotional distress.

The good news is that there are a lot of treatment strategies are available. The sooner the treatment is initiated, lower the risk for lasting emotional and physical damage.

The Symptoms of Acne

Acne usually develops on shoulders, back, chest, neck and face, which are the parts of the skin with the biggest number of functional oil glands. Acne vulgaris can take the following forms:

1. Inflammatory lesions

- Cysts – are sore, pus-loaded lumps underneath the skin surface. Cysts are similar to boils which can result to scarring.

- Nodules – are solid, sore and large lumps underneath the skin's surface. They are formed by the accumulation of secretions deep within the hair follicles.

- Pimples or pustule - are tender and red bumps which are filled with white pus at their tips

- Papules – are tiny raised bumps that indicate the presence of an infection or inflammation in the hair follicles. Papules may be tender and appear red.

2. Non-Inflammatory Lesions

- Whiteheads or blackheads (comedones) – are formed when the openings of the hair follicles get plugged and blocked with dead skin cells, oil, and sometimes bacteria. Comedones that are open and appear dark are called blackheads. Comedones that are closed and appear as slightly raised, skin-colored lumps are called whiteheads.

Know When to See your Physician

Acne vulgaris is not a life-threatening health condition, although you may wish to get medical advice from a skin specialist for inflamed cysts to prevent scarring or other lasting damages to the skin.

If your acne condition and the scars that it may have left are affecting your self-esteem or social relationships, you may also seek the advice of your dermatologist. Ask if your acne can be controlled or if there is something that may be done to remove (or at least lighten) the scars.

The Causes of Acne

The following factors contribute to the development of acne:

- Accumulation of bacteria
- Irregular shedding of dead skin cells leading to the irritation of the skin's hair follicles
- Overproduction of oil (sebum)

Acne takes place when the skin's hair follicles become clogged up with dead skin cells and oil. The skin's hair follicles are linked to the sebaceous glands. These glands are responsible for synthesizing an oily substance commonly known as sebum to lubricate your skin and hair.

Oil is usually transported up along the hair shafts then out through the pores of the skin's hair follicles and into the skin surface. When the body synthesizes excessive amounts of sebum and sheds too much dead skin cells, these two accumulate in the hair follicles and develop together as a soft plug – a good environment where bacterial organisms can live.

This plug may make the hair follicle wall to swell and create a whitehead. The plug may also be open to the skin surface and may appear dark resulting to a blackhead. Pimples are slightly raised spots which appear red with a white center. They form when microbes attack clogged hair follicles.

Inflammation and blockages that develop deep inside hair follicles creates lumps underneath the skin surface called cysts. Other skin pores, which are the openings of the sweat gland found on the skin, are not usually involved in acne condition.

Factors that May Aggravate Acne

The following are some of the known factors that can worsen or trigger an existing case of acne:

- Diet – recent research indicates that some dietary factors (such as consuming too much carbohydrate-rich foods and dairy products) can increase blood sugar levels, which in turn may trigger the development of acne lesions.

- Certain Medications – medications which contain lithium, androgens and corticosteroids are known to cause acne.

- Hormones – androgens are specific types of hormones that increase in levels during adolescence, forcing the sebaceous glands to enlarge and produce more sebum. Hormonal changes brought about by the use of oral contraceptives, as well as pregnancy, also have an impact on sebum production.

Risk Factors of Acne

Hormonal changes in the body can worsen or trigger acne. Such hormonal changes are commonly observed in:

- Individuals using certain types of drugs, such as those containing lithium, androgens or corticosteroids
- Pregnant women

- Girls and women, two to seven days prior their periods

Other risk factors of acne include:

- Stress (does not cause acne, although if you already have acne, stress can actually make it worse)

- Pressure or friction on the skin (brought about by different items such as backpacks, tight collars, helmets, cellphones or telephones)

- Family history of acne (if your parents have suffered from acne, then you are likely to have acne as well)

- Direct skin contact (with oily or greasy substances or with specific types of cosmetics)

2: Foods to Eat and Foods to Avoid

In 2010, a group of researchers have surprised a lot of people when they reported that the food that we eat can have an impact on acne outbreaks. That same year, an article in the scientific journal "Skin Therapy Letter" highlighted the outcomes of an analysis conducted with 27 samples.

The experts reported that the consumption of cow's milk increased acne severity and prevalence. They also discovered an association between acne risk and glycemic index. In an earlier study published in 2007, similar results have been obtained. Experts from Australia reported that young males aged 15 to 25 with mild to moderate cases of acne have experienced drastic improvements when they shifted from consuming the usual American diet (composed of white bread and severely processed breakfast cereals) to a healthier one composed of vegetables, fruits, lean meat and whole grains.

The experts from the Royal Melbourne Institute of Technology in Australia reported that the acne of the boys on the low-glycemic index and higher protein diet significantly improved by 50 percent, which is actually even more than what is commonly achieved with topical acne treatments.

Some individuals have believed for many years that diet can affect acne, although only recently have scientific experts started to discover evidence that this hypothesis is indeed true.

Type of Foods to Avoid

Recent studies have been focused on the foods that can aggravate acne. The following are some food items that come up most usually as culprits in encouraging acne breakouts. Stay away from these food items and see if you will notice an improvement.

1. Fast Food

   Oily fast food causes inflammations in the body. Researchers have already associated fast foods to health conditions (such as asthma) strictly due to its ability to increase the overall inflammation in the body. Inflammations can also cause acne breakouts; so if you are dining in a fast-food joint, go for the salad or yogurt.

2. Junk food

   Due to their ability to increase blood sugar levels and induce hormonal fluctuations, junk foods are on the stay-away-from list if you are trying to clear up your skin.

3. High-glycemic foods

   These are the types of food that tend to break down rapidly in the body, promoting the increase of insulin levels and raising the levels of blood sugar. High-glycemic foods can promote inflammation and hormonal fluctuations – both can trigger an acne breakout. High glycemic foods include cakes, cookies, potato chips, pretzels, white rice, processed breakfast cereals and white bread. Instead of eating those, go for low glycemic-index foods such as sweet potatoes, whole grains, vegetables and most type of fruits.

4. Sugar

   You may have long suspected that sugar is associated with acne flare-ups. Some studies currently suggest that there could be an association. This does not imply however, that if you munch on a cookie, you will get a pimple. It boils down to the amount of sugar that you're eating in a day.

   If you take in a candy bar and a can of soda for instance, you are most likely causing a spike to your blood sugar levels and you may experience acne breakouts after a few hours. If you think that sugar is causing your acne breakouts, cut back on your sugar intake and see if you experience any difference.

5. Cow's milk

According to the study conducted in 2010, there is a link between drinking cow's milk and acne. The experts remain unsure why this could be the case, although there are a number of different theories. Cow's milk tends to increase blood sugar levels, which in turn boosts inflammation (causing pimple breakouts). It can also raise insulin levels, which promotes the production of sebum (skin oil).

Majority of milk products available in the market comes from pregnant cows, and hence contain other hormones that can promote the production of sebum. Milk also contains growth hormones which can promote the overgrowth of skin cells, leading to clogged pores.

In the year 2005, experts conducted a study and found out that participants who consume more milk during their teenage years had much higher rates of severe acne than those who drank little to no milk during their teenage years.

The Truth about Acne and Chocolates

Chocolate has been long alleged to be causing acne, although recently it has received a pass. In one small study conducted in 2013 in Netherlands, experts discovered an association between eating chocolates and skin changes resulting to acne. For the study, the researchers gathered blood samples from 7 healthy individuals before and after they consumed chocolate daily for 4 days.

The researchers then exposed the blood samples to Propionibacterium acnes (the bacterial organisms which contribute to acne when they thrive inside the blocked skin pores) and to staphylococcus aureus (which is another skin bacteria that can make acne worse).

The blood samples from the participants (after eating chocolate) synthesized more interleukin-1b which is an indicator for inflammation after exposure to Propionibacterium acnes.

Consuming chocolates also boosted the synthesis of interleukin 10, another immune system factor, after being exposed to Staphylococcus aureus. Interleukin 10 is believed to reduce the body's natural defenses against pathogenic microorganisms, so increased levels could let the bacteria to infect the pimples and make them even worse.

This indicates that eating chocolate could promote inflammation and bacterial infection, making acne even worse. As this is only a small study, more research is required.

Dark chocolate contains health-promoting antioxidants; so based on how much chocolate you consume each day, you may want to wait for further evidence. In the meantime, to find out if your skin is sensitive to chocolate, try avoiding it for an entire week and see if you can observe any significant improvements on your skin's condition.

Foods to Eat to Achieve Acne-Free Skin

Just staying away from the acne-promoting foods mentioned above will likely to lead to acne-free skin, particularly if you were eating them regularly before. But what if you are already following a healthy diet?

Are there certain types of foods that would provide you with the edge against acne break outs? Scientific studies are in the earliest stages, although we have some knowledge of certain foods that could be beneficial. The following are some of them:

1. Probiotics

Probiotics have been discovered to lessen inflammation in the gut, which may eventually help to reduce acne break outs. Based on a study conducted in 2011, the microflora in the intestines may have an impact on inflammation throughout the body, which in turn, can affect acne flare ups.

Prior studies indicate that patients suffering from acne were more likely to manifest response to bacterial strains obtained from stool. In other words, toxic materials from the gut were a key feature in the acne condition. Because pre- and probiotics can lessen both oxidative stress and inflammation, experts claim that they may help lessen acne breakouts.

This seems to be more than sufficient proof to say that microorganisms in the gut, as well as the integrity of the gastrointestinal tract itself, are key factors in having acne breakouts. To obtain more probiotics in your diet, try eating kombucha tea, kimchi, tempeh, pickles, miso soup, microalgae, dark chocolate, sauerkraut, kefir and yogurt.

2. Juicing

Vegetables and fruits can help to naturally clear up acne. A lot contain beta-carotenes, which naturally help lessen the production of sebum and all have anti-inflammatory properties. Leafy, dark green vegetables can also help flush out the toxic materials from the body which promote acne flare ups. Dark-colored berries also contain phytonutrients which are good for skin health.

3. Oysters

Many studies show that the mineral zinc may lessen the effects of acne. It is more advisable to obtain zinc from food, because too much zinc from supplements (over 100mg daily) can trigger adverse side effects. Consume more oysters, dried watermelon seeds, squash seeds, roasted pumpkin seeds, roast beef, veal liver and toasted wheat germ (sprinkled on steamed veggies and salads).

4. Green tea

Studies have indicated that green tea helps combat acne. Researchers from South Korea have found out that applying creams which contain EGCG (a potent antioxidant found in green tea) lessen the size of the sebaceous glands, which are typically enlarged in individuals suffering from acne.

A follow-up study also indicated that EGCG lessened sebum production. A study involving human participants revealed that EGCG drastically improves skin condition, effectively alleviating acne symptoms. Consume more green tea through the entire day and try directly applying cooled tea bags to acne-prone areas of the face for about 15 minutes.

5. Flax or flaxseed

The usual Western diet is composed of excessive amounts of omega-6 fatty acids, which are associated with inflammation. Consuming more omega-3 fatty acids, such as those that are found in flaxseed, walnuts, and fatty fish, can help reduce inflammation and improve acne flare-ups.

3: Sample Acne-Free Menu Plan

Only foods with considerable carbohydrate content have an effect on the blood sugar levels. The Glycemic Index (GI) is a measure of how much a certain food item influences blood sugar levels. Its value is computed for in relation to a 50-gram serving of carbohydrate.

Foods with high GI (having scores of over 70) include biscuits, potatoes, white bread and sugary ready-to-eat breakfast cereals. These foods are rapidly broken down and absorbed in the blood stream, which leads blood sugar levels to spike instantaneously.

This spike in blood sugar levels prompts the pancreas to synthesize high amounts of insulin, which stimulates the hormones that are linked with acne. Foods with low GI (having scores below 55) include baked beans, basmati rice, wholegrain bread and porridge; these are ingested and absorbed slowly, causing the blood sugar levels to increase slowly over time and induce a milder insulin reaction. Choosing healthier carbohydrates is the key to acne-free skin.

That's why you need to learn about the differences between the conventional Western diet and the anti-acne diet. You'll also have to know which food items have low GI values.

Western Diet vs. Anti-Acne Diet

Western Diet	Anti-Acne Diet
Soft Drinks	Fruit juice, low-fat milk, water
Potatoes	Carrots, sweet corn or sweet potatoes
Crisps	Plain popcorn
Muesli bars, lollies, cakes, biscuits	Low-fat dairy products, seeds, unsalted nuts, dried fruits, vegetables and fresh fruits
Sugar	Honey
Crackers	Grainy crisp breads
White rice	Fresh noodles, pasta, doongara rice or basmati rice
Whole meal or white bread	Fruit loaf, sourdough bread, grainy bread
Sugary ready-to-eat breakfast cereals	Natural muesli, rolled oats, high-fiber breakfast cereals

Examples of Low Glycemic Index (GI) Foods

Food Items	GI Value
Meat, Seafood and Protein	
Veal, lean	0

Lamb, lean	0
Fish	0
Eggs	0
Skinless Chicken	0
Lean Beef	0
Dairy Products	
Skim Milk	32
Reduced-fat custard	37
Low-fat vanilla ice cream	46
Low-fat yogurt	33
Low-fat chocolate milk	34
Pasta and Noodles	
Vermicelli	35
Spaghetti	44
Macaroni	47
Lasagna	53
Fresh Rice Noodles	40
Beans and Legumes	
Red Kidney Beans	37
Four Bean Mix	36
Chickpeas	28
Baked Beans	49
Vegetables	
Zucchini	0
Tomato	0
Sweet corn	46
Squash	0
Spinach	0

Snow pea sprouts	0
Onions	0
Mushrooms	0
Lettuce	0
Cucumber	0
Celery	0
Cauliflower	0
Carrot	41
Capsicum	0
Broccoli	0
Asparagus	0
Fruit Juices	
Pineapple juice	46
Unsweetened freshly squeezed orange juice	50
Cranberry juice	52
Unsweetened Apple juice	40
Canned Fruit with Natural Juices	
Pear	44
Peach	45
Dried Fruits	
Prunes	29
Apricots	30
Apple	29
Fresh Fruits	
Strawberries	40
Plum	39
Pear	38

Peach	42
Orange	42
Mango	51
Kiwi Fruit	53
Grapes	53
Banana	52
Apple	38

The best way to get rid of acne is through having a healthy eating plan which includes low GI carbohydrates and protein-rich foods. The following is a recommended 2-week anti-acne menu which features a vast assortment of healthy recipes (do keep in mind that most of these recipes don't come with specific cooking instructions since they're basically modified versions of easy-to-prepare classics, such as salads, sandwiches, and omelets):

Week 1

Day	Breakfast	Lunch	Dinner
1	2 slices of spice and fruit toast with a teaspoon of margarine 1 pc of fresh fruit 1 glass of low-fat milk	Chicken and pasta salad (100 grams of skinless chicken, ¾ cup of cooked pasta, a cup of salad vegetables, and a tbsp. oil-free dressing)	Garlic and Oregano Roast Lamb plus 1 and a half cup of roasted vegetables Dessert: 2 scoops of low-fat ice-cream with 1 small bowl of fresh fruit salad
2	Cinnamon-Ricotta Toast (2 pieces of wholegrain toast, 40 grams of low-fat ricotta cheese, cinnamon,	Spinach, sweet corn and mushroom omelet (½ cup of spinach, ½ cup of mushrooms, ½ cup sweet corn,	Steak Sandwich 1 tbsp. oil-free dressing ½ cups of salad vegetables Dessert: A bowl of stewed fruit

	and a dab of honey) A piece of fresh fruit	40 grams low-fat grated cheddar cheese, and 2 eggs)	

| 3 | Sautéed tomato and mushrooms 2 slices of wholegrain toast with a teaspoon of margarine Slices of fresh fruit | Salmon and salad sandwich (40 grams of low-fat cheese, half a cup of salad vegetables, 2 slices wholegrain bread, and 100 grams of salmon) | Mediterranean Feta Lamb Chops (Grill a bunch of asparagus and 150 grams of lean lamb chops with olive oil and lemon juice. Drizzle low-fat feta and scatter cherry tomatoes over the lamb chops. Serve with a cup of mixed salad greens.) Dessert: a small bowl of fresh fruit salad |
| 4 | Sautéed tomato and mushrooms 2 pieces of wholegrain | Turkey and mayo pita (1 tbsp. low-fat mayonnaise, | Grilled Calamari (Grill 150 grams calamari and |

toast with a teaspoon of margarine 250 grams of low-fat yogurt	½ cup of salad greens, 100 grams lean turkey, and 1 whole meal pita bread)	serve with a 2 cups of salad vegetables and a tablespoon of dressing – balsamic vinegar, olive oil, and garlic) Dessert: A small bowl of stewed fruit, unsweetened

5	A piece of fresh fruit ½ cup of low-fat yogurt ¾ cups of high-fiber breakfast cereal with half a cup of low-fat milk	Ham and mustard sandwich 1 teaspoon mustard 100 grams lean ham 2 pieces of wholegrain bread ½ cup of salad	Vietnamese Beef and Glass Noodle Salad Dessert: 2 scoops of low-fat ice cream served with a small bowl of peaches
6	1 fruit smoothie (Prepared by Blending together a piece of fresh fruit, half a cup of low-fat milk, 1 teaspoon of honey, and half a tub of low-fat yogurt.)	Rare roast beef with salad wrap (1 tablespoon of sweet chili sauce, ½ cup of salad greens, 100 grams lean rare roast beef, 1 piece pita bread) A piece of fresh fruit	Grill snapper (Serve 150 grams of grilled snapper with olive oil, ginger and garlic, together with 2 cups of steamed veggies.) Dessert: 200 grams of low-fat custard with a

	2 pieces boiled eggs		small bowl of diet jelly
7	1 small can of baked beans served with 2 pieces of wholegrain toast A glass of low-fat milk with cocoa	Lamb salad (1 tablespoon oil-free dressing, 1 cup of salad greens, and 100g diced lean lamb) A piece of fresh fruit	Tandoori chicken strips (150 grams of skinless chicken strips prepared in tandoori sauce with a cup of veggies. Serve with ¾ cup of steamed basmati rice) Dessert: 200 grams of low-fat yoghurt served with a small bowl of stewed unsweetened fruit.
Snacks	Fruit • 159 grams of canned fruit, in natural	Low-fat Dairy • 200 ml of low-fat drinking yogurt	Low Glycemic Index Carbohydrates • 1 cup of unsalted and

	juices • 30 g of dried fruit such as prunes, pears, peaches, apple and apricots • 1 pc of fresh fruit	• 200 g of low-fat frozen yogurt • 200g of low-fat yogurt	plain popcorn • 2 slices of spice and fruit toast • 30 grams or a handful of nuts

Week 2

Day	Breakfast	Lunch	Dinner
1	2 pieces of wholegrain toast, 1 tomato, half a cup of baby spinach leaves, 2 poached eggs and a teaspoon of margarine. 1 piece of fresh fruit 1 glass of skimmed milk	Tuna and four-bean salad (Prepared with 1 tablespoon of oil-free dressing, 100 grams tuna, and a cup of four-bean mix. Serve with 1 piece of wholegrain roll.) Dessert: 200 grams of low-fat yogurt	Lemon and Rosemary Lamb Kebabs (Thread red onion wedges and 150 grams of diced lean lamb fillets on skewers, brush with olive oil, rosemary, lemon rind and juice and garlic. Barbecue and serve with a cup of salad greens and a tablespoon of balsamic vinegar.) Dessert:

			Low-fat yogurt with a small bowl of fruit salad

2	200 grams of low-fat berry yogurt served with 150 grams of mixed berries	Turkey roll (100 grams of lean turkey, 1 tablespoon of cranberry sauce, a slice of low-fat Swiss cheese, and half a cup of salad greens rolled into a piece of wholegrain bread.)	Spaghetti Bolognese ser6ved with 1 and a half cup of salad greens with a tablespoon of oil-free dressing. Dessert: A piece of fresh fruit
3	1 piece of fresh fruit 1 cup of skimmed milk ¾ cups of high-fiber breakfast cereal	Egg and Salad Sandwich (½ cup of salad greens, 2 tablespoons of low-fat mayonnaise, 2 pieces hard boiled eggs, and 2	2 cups of steamed vegetables 150 grams of barbecued salmon Dessert: 2 cups of low-fat ice cream served with a small bowl of

		pieces whole grain bread)	pears

4	1 teaspoon of passion fruit pulp, 5 pieces strawberries 200 grams of low-fat vanilla yogurt ¾ cup natural untoasted muesli	Chicken Greek salad (40 grams of low-fat feta cheese, 2 teaspoon of olive oil, 1 tablespoon of balsamic vinegar, 1 cup of salad vegetables and 100 grams of grilled skinless chicken breast served with a piece of whole meal pita bread.)	Herb-crusted Lamb cutlets served with half a cup of roasted vegetables Dessert: A small bowl of unsweetened stewed fruit
5	1 fresh fruit smoothie (prepared by blending a teaspoon of honey, ½ tub of low-	Cheese, tomato and ham roll (½ cup of shredded lettuce, 1 piece	Creamy Beef Stroganoff served with ¾ cup of steamed basmati rice and 1 and a

fat yogurt, half a cup of low-fat milk and a piece of fresh fruit)	tomato, 1 tablespoon, chutney, 100 grams lean ham, a slice of low-fat cheddar cheese – all wrapped in wholegrain roll)	half cup of steamed vegetables Dessert: 200 grams of low-fat yogurt with a small bowl of stewed fruit

6	2 pieces of whole grain toast with vegemite and 1 teaspoon margarine 1 piece fresh fruit A glass of low-fat milk	Roast Lamb Wrap (Half a cup of tabbouleh, a tablespoon of hummus, and 100 grams of leftover lamb wrapped in 1 whole meal pita bread)	Baked Chicken with Thyme (Bake 150 grams of skinless chicken breast fillets with olive oil, lemon juice, thyme and rosemary. Serve with ½ cups of steamed veggies and half a cup of roasted sweet potato) Dessert: 200 grams of low-fat custard with a small bowl or peaches
7	200 grams low-fat yogurt with	Avocado, salmon and salad	Tuna Pasta (1 tablespoon of olive oil,

| | a small bowl of fresh fruit salad | sandwich (½ cup of salad vegetables, avocado, 100 grams of salmon, and 2 pieces of wholegrain bread) | 2 tablespoon of tomato paste, 1 and a half cup of vegetables such as asparagus, zucchini, tomatoes, and 150 grams tuna – all tossed in with ¾ cups of cooked pasta)

Dessert:
A small bowl of fresh fruit salad |
| Snacks | Fruits
• 150 grams of canned fruit
• 30 grams of | Low-Fat Dairy Products
• 1 mug of hot chocolate prepared | Low GI Carbohydrates
• A handful or 30 grams of nuts
• 2 pieces wholegr |

		dried fruits such as prunes, pears, peaches, apple and apricots • 1 piece of fresh fruit	with 1 teaspoon of cocoa and 250 ml low-fat milk • 200 grams of low-fat custard with diet jelly • 250 ml low-fat milk	ain toast/bread or 2 grainy crisp breads with vegetable soup, baked beans, hummus or vegemite

To improve your intake of protein-rich foods and low Glycemic Index carbohydrates, follow these tips:

1. Have an Oil Change

- Add avocado to a salad or a sandwich

- Sprinkle seeds and nuts on cereals
- Go for monosaturated margarine
- Use olive and canola oil in cooking

2. Get fresh

- Consume about 2 and a half vegetables daily, ideally the non-starchy varieties such as capsicum and broccoli which have a lower GI value

- Go for three servings of fruit every day

3. Minimize Processed Foods

- Reduce refined white foods such as biscuits, cakes and bread
- Keep fast meal options at home to avoid the need of having fast food delivered
- Instead of drinking soda, drink water
- Stay away from sugary breakfast cereals as well as ready-to-eat snacks

4. Go low GI

   To make sure that your carbohydrate choices are of the low Glycemic Index kind, keep these in mind:

- Add chickpeas, lentils, tofu and legumes to salads and stews

- Instead of white rice, select basmati rice and pasta
- Switch from white bread to rye and wholegrain varieties
- Begin your day with high fiber breakfast cereals such as wheat biscuits, natural muesli or porridge

5. Power up with Protein

- Go for three servings of low-fat dairy products daily
- Consume lean protein such as fish, poultry or red meat for lunch every day
- Include eggs in your meals from time to time
- Incorporate lean veal, lamb or beef at least thrice a week
- Have fish for dinner twice a week

Tips When Eating Out

Consuming healthy meals is usually a lot easier during the weekdays, when there is a set routine; although it can get challenging during the weekends when teenagers are out with their friends or the entire family dines out.

This is why it is so essential that you understand how to make healthy food choices to stay free from acne.

The following are some basic healthy food rules that you must follow to stay acne-free:

- Stay away from certain add-ons such as white bread rolls and fries, and instead go for side salads or steamed vegetables

- Minimize dishes that are crumbed, battered, pan-fried or deep-fried
- Request dressings and sauces to be put on the side and use only a little
- Finish your meal with skimmed hot chocolate instead of sugar-loaded desserts

Tips When Eating Out to Stay Acne-Free

Type of Cuisine	Choose	Limit
Chinese	Steamed appetizers Clear soups Steamed rice and stir fries with seafood, chicken, lamb,	Toast and prawn crackers Deep-fried foods such as fried ice cream, dim

	beef, tofu and vegetables	sums, egg rolls and spring rolls Lemon-sauce or sweet and sour dishes

Japanese	Udon or teriyaki noodles in broth Ramen noodle dishes Miso soup Sashimi and sushi	Deep fried dishes such as tempura (vegetables or seafood in batter) or katsudon (fried pork chop)
Vietnamese	Pho (rice noodle soup served with lean pieces of chicken and beef with limes, chili and bean shoots) Other excellent choices include Vietnamese rice paper rolls, stir fries and steamed rice	Fried noodle dishes and spring rolls
Thai	Hot pots, Thai beef salad Satay skweres Stir-fries	Fried noodles such as pad thai Coconut-based

	Tom Yum Goong	curries Deep fried entrees such as fish cakes

Indian	Rogan josh (goat or lamb in tomato sauce Yogurt-based curries Dishes with lentils Chickpeas with vegetables Tandoori Steamed basmati rice	Butter sauces Creamy curries such as korma Oily breads such as naan Pappadams Curry puffs Fried samosas
Italian	Pasta with tomato sauces such as Bolognese and Minestrone Sorbet or fresh fruit for dessert	Extra parmesan cheese Fried mozzarella sticks Garlic bread Creamy pasta sauces or risottos such as boscaiola Lasagna
Greek	Grilled seafood or lamb dishes	Fried foods such as baklava or

	Dolmades (stuffed vie leave) served with Greek salad	calamari Cheese dishes such as moussaka

4: Natural Supplements to Boost your Acne

A study conducted at the University of Miami whose outcomes were published at the annual meeting of the American Academy of Dermatology in 2009 revealed that a low-carbohydrate diet, also commonly referred to as low-glycemic diet, results in reduced acne severity and incidence.

The experts concluded that lifestyle factors, such as diet, can play a crucial role in the skin's overall health. To further boost the anti-acne properties of your acne-free diet, it is recommended that you supplement with the following acne-fighting nutrients and herbs:

Nutritional Supplements:

1. Vitamin A

Vitamin A is a natural antioxidant that belongs to family of substances commonly referred to as retinoids. Retinol is the term used to describe the active alcohol form of vitamin A. Vitamin A has been prescribed for many years by dermatologists to naturally treat acne lesions.

Low levels of vitamin A in the body have been linked with inflammation and acne. This vitamin is responsible for normal vision, healthy skin, immune system support, red blood cell production and overall growth and development of the body. Food sources of vitamin A include cod liver oils, spinach, sweet potatoes, as well as yellow and orange fruits and vegetables.

Vitamin A is crucial for the normal shedding of dead skin cells that accumulate inside the skin's pores. Vitamin A helps to prevent excessive accumulation that would otherwise result to a clogged skin pore. Furthermore, the anti-oxidant properties of this vitamin serves as an anti-inflammatory for the skin and helps to calm sore, red and swollen acne lesions.

It is highly suggested that persons suffering from inflammatory acne on the body and/or the face consume foods that are rich in vitamin A and supplement with 10,000 IU of vitamin A every day. If you are pregnant, it is advised that you seek medical clearance before you start supplementing with vitamin A.

2. Selenium

Selenium is an essential mineral that possesses anti-oxidant properties. It is also capable of boosting the effectiveness of other antioxidative substances. Selenium can be found in halibut, seafood salmon, nuts and grains.

To be a bit more specific, selenium has been found to work in synergy with, as well as preserve the integrity of, other types of antioxidants such as zinc. This mineral works in glutathione peroxidase, which is a type of enzyme that is very crucial in the prevention of acne inflammation.

Minute amounts of selenium, and vitamin E have been indicated to help improve acne, specifically in patients with low baseline glutathione enzyme activity. Furthermore, studies indicate that a deficiency in selenium may have a crucial role in inflammatory conditions such as psoriasis, eczema and acne.

This mineral must be consumed along with other types of antioxidants as well as zinc supplements. The recommended daily dose is 48 micrograms.

3. Zinc

Zinc is a type of mineral that plays a crucial role in a lot of bodily functions including immune system function, reproduction, brain function and growth and development. Excellent sources of zinc include oysters, lean meats, whole grains, oatmeal, seeds, nuts and beans.

This mineral has a lot of crucial functions for acne treatment. First, zinc helps in the metabolism of essential omega 3 fatty acids.

Secondly, it is an essential anti-inflammatory and antioxidant. Third, it aids in breaking down substance P, which is a nerve substance that promotes sebum synthesis when the body is under duress. Fourth, this mineral is responsible for transporting vitamin A, which is a natural anti-acne vitamin, from the liver. Current studies show that individuals suffering from acne have low levels of zinc in their body.

4. Omega-3 fatty Acids

Eicosapentaenoic Acid or simply EPA is a type of omega-3 fatty acid which is found in seafood, specifically fatty, ocean fish such as anchovies, sardines and mackerel. EPA is undoubtedly the most excellent anti-inflammatory found in nature.

Inflammation is at the core of the acne condition, both systemically and externally. Thus, a potent anti-inflammatory supplement is the key to successfully treating acne. The process of inflammation is prompted at the systemic level and then, along with other key factors, results to the formation of acne at the skin level. Inflammation is also associated with most chronic illnesses such as arthritis, heart diseases and diabetes.

Omega-3 fatty acids help clear acne lesions by inhibiting 2 inflammatory substances that contribute to acne flare-ups. These two substances are called LTB4 and PGE2. According to experts, individuals with diets high in omega-3 fatty acids (such people in Papua New Guinea, the coastal regions of North Carolina, and in Japan) all have low incidence of acne.

It is highly suggested that individuals suffering from inflammatory acne on the face and/or the body must consume foods that are abundant in omega-3 fatty acids. It might also be necessary to start taking 2,000 milligrams of EPA omega-3 each day.

Make sure to check the labels of your supplements as you want to have a minimum of 1,000 milligrams of EPA each day. If you are pregnant, it is best to consult with your physician before you start supplementing with EPA.

In addition to supplements, fatty fishes such as mackerel, sardines and anchovies, as well as healthy oils including canola, walnut and flax oil are excellent sources of essential omega-3 fatty acids. Eating imega-3 fortified eggs would also prove to be beneficial. Palm, sunflower, peanut, soybean as well as other vegetable oils must be strictly avoided as they tend to aggravate acne by prompting the secretion of PGE2 (which, as mentioned, is a substance that causes acne).

Herbal Supplements

1. Vitex

   Some females experience acne breakouts at certain times during their menstrual cycle. It is highly recommended for them to take about 40 drops of vitex extract or a capsule made from the dried plant daily. Vitex is a type of fruiting tree which is grown in the Mediterranean areas. Vitex has long been utilized to help alleviate pre-menstrual symptoms due to its apparent ability to stimulate progesterone. If you are nursing or pregnant, do not take vitex.

2. Dandelion

   The leaves of dandelion have a lot of advantageous properties. This includes stimulating the liver, which is the body's primary filtering organ. The dandelion's root possesses anti-inflammatory properties and is packed with vitamins including vitamin E, which aids in maintaining the skin's overall health. Prepare tea from dried dandelion leaves or roots.

3. Burdock

Burdock is an herb which resembles Velcro due to its prickly, hooked balls. Burdock is frequently utilized in Asian cuisine, specifically in some types of sushi. This herb is a diuretic which encourages urination and sweating, which triggers the body to release waste materials including the fatty acid synthesized by the bacteria P. acnes. Search for Burdock root in Asian groceries and prepare a tea with a teaspoon of dried root steeped in about 2 cups of hot water. Sip up to 4 cups of tea prepared from Burdock each day and enjoy acne-free skin.

5: Common Myths about Acne and the Truth behind Them

Even though you already know a lot about the best ways of fighting acne, it'd still be beneficial for you to discover the truth on some common myths about the dermal dilemma.

Acne Myth No.1:
Adults do not develop acne

According to major surveys, a considerable number of adults still develop acne in their 30's or 40's. Some even develop acne during their 50s. Adult acne is more likely to appear as red nodules found around the jaw and mouth, rather than emerge in the form of blackheads and whiteheads found all over the cheeks, nose and forehead.

Acne Myth No. 2:
Stress can result to the development of acne

This acne myth is actually true, but knowing the extent at which stress affects the skin condition is definitely hard. After all, there are several studies that seem to indicate that college students have increased acne flare-ups during their finals.

Acne Myth No.3:
Sunscreen can make your acne worse so stay away from using them

The key is to choose the right type of sunscreen. Certain sunscreens disperse UV light with the use of a chemical reaction. This may lead to the formation of heat bumps. If your skin is acne-pone, use physical sunscreens such as those that contain zinc oxide.

Acne Myth No. 4:
Acne develops on your skin because you are not washing it enough

This is not probably true, unless you are a slob. Clinical studies involving teenagers show that washing the face two times daily is more effective that just doing it only once, although anything more than that is not necessary. In fact, excessive washing may even dry the skin, making it much more prone to acne.

Acne Myth No. 5:
You cannot wear makeup if you have an acne breakout

Certain types of makeup can certainly make acne worse, specifically thick liquid foundations and stage-type pancake makeup. Applying looser and lighter powder foundations (such as mineral foundations) probably wouldn't worsen your acne. Also, do keep in mind that there are products specifically made for covering acne.

Acne Myth No. 6:

Acne is just a cosmetic problem
Acne can have long-lasting effects in how you feel about yourself and if improperly managed or left untreated, it can lead to permanent scarring of the skin.

Acne Myth No. 7:

You just have to wait and just allow acne to fade away with time

That's definitely a bad idea. There are a lot of treatments available and dermatologists can help you in finding the most suitable treatment strategy. There are also some dietary changes (such as the one you've just read about) that you might like to try. See if you can get amazing results from them.

Acne Myth No.8:

You can clean up a pimple by thoroughly scrubbing it

Scrubbing your acne thoroughly is actually the worst thing that you can do. Also, those who spend hours popping their pimples will surely regret doing it. Applying excessive amounts of pressure to irritated skin is among the best ways to get a scar. If you have big acne lesions and you have a big date today, you may opt to get a pimple injection from your dermatologist that will lessen its size and reduce the inflammation.

Acne Myth No.9:
You can go to the cosmetics section and get yourself an excellent cleanser of face cream

Individuals will find their way to the department store and seek recommendations from the person selling beauty products, although they will not go to an expert who could give real sound advice for their skin condition. Simply put, relying on cheap creams and cleansers often leads to disappointment.

Acne Myth No. 10:
Sex can cause acne

The truth of the matter is that, the sex hormone, commonly referred to as androgens (hormones that are produced during adolescence period) has been associated with cases of acne. However, while this hormone, as well as other types of hormones, triggers a stronger sex drive, there has been no clear proof that sexual engagements and masturbation can make acne even worse.

Acne Myth No. 11:
Exposure to sun can help treat acne

While the sun's rays can give a short-term fix to conceal the appearance of acne, it isn't capable of curing the skin condition. What the sun really provides is some sort of camouflage that blends the skin tone with the acne marks. Excessive exposure to the sun does not only lead to dryness and irritation, but it also makes your skin more prone to cancer, premature aging and sunburns. Be sure to always use a non-comedogenic sunscreen to help safeguard your skin.

Conclusion

I hope this book was able to help you to have a better understanding of acne, its causes, risk factors and symptoms.

The next step is to try the simple dietary tips and follow the anti-acne diet menu plan so that you'd finally bid your acne goodbye. Also, don't forget to try supplementing with some of the most potent vitamins, minerals, and herbs to stay acne-free forever.

Finally, if you enjoyed this book, please take the time to share your thoughts and post a review. It'd be greatly appreciated!